THE SIRTFOOD
COOKBOOK

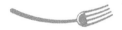

*Delicious Recipes
for Your Sirtfood Diet*

CATHERINE MILLER

Special Edition Recipes

—

TABLE OF CONTENTS

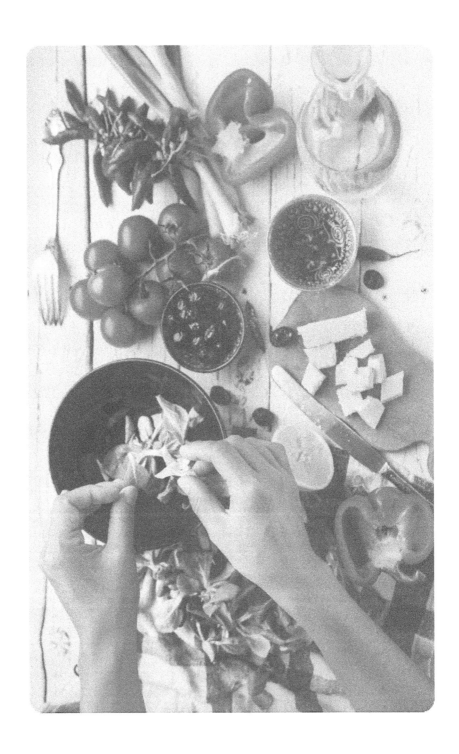

Introduction

Thank you for purchasing this book.

If you are familiar with the Sirtfood Diet, you are surely looking for recipes to help you carry on this diet.

Let's remember now the main points of this diet.

The Sirtfood Diet is based on a group of nutrients capable of activating a family of genes existing in each of us: the sirtuins. They can stimulate the metabolism and activate the "thinness gene," which is combined with meat and fish, to be consumed every day by drastically reducing the number of carbohydrates and total daily calories.

Among these foods, we generally consider about twenty, called the "top Sitfoods."

Top 20 Sirt foods

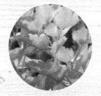
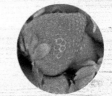

1. Buckwheat
2. Capers
3. Celery
4. Chilli pepper
5. Cocoa
6. Coffee
7. Cabbage
8. Extra virgin olive oil
9. Lovage or mountain celery
10. Matcha Green Tea
11. Medjool Dates
12. Parsley
13. Red chicory
14. Red onion
15. Red wine
16. Rocket salad
17. Soy
18. Strawberries
19. Walnuts
20. Turmeric

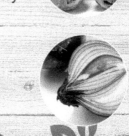

The TOP Sirtfoods

1. Buckwheat
2. Capers
3. Celery
4. Chilli pepper, especially the bird's-eye chilli
5. Cocoa
6. Coffee
7. Cabbage
8. Extra virgin olive oil
9. Lovage or mountain celery
10. Matcha Green Tea
11. Medjool Dates
12. Parsley
13. Red chicory
14. Red onion
15. Red wine
16. Rocket salad
17. Soy
18. Strawberries
19. Walnuts
20. Turmeric

Diet Plan

The **First Phase** lasts <u>one week</u>.

During the first 3 days, the meal plan is as follows:

> *3 green juices Sirt*
>
> *+ 1 solid meal*
>
> *+ 15-20g of dark chocolate*

While, from day 4 to day 7, it is:

> *2 green Sirt juices*
>
> *+ 2 solid meals*
>
> *+ 15-20g of dark chocolate*

***

The **Second Phase** of the diet lasts <u>two weeks</u> and consolidates the weight loss achieved in the first.

> *1 green Sirt juices*
>
> *+ 3 solid meal*
>
> *+ 15-20g dark chocolate*

The Green Juice

The green Sirtfood Diet juice is the *central* piece of the Sirtfood diet.

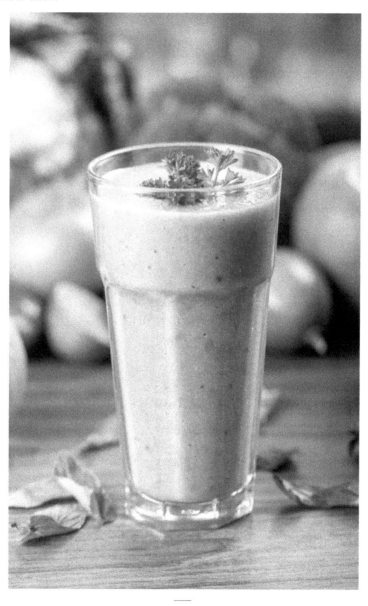

Whether you are not aiming to follow the diet, the liquid is full of nutrients and a great choice for a regular diet. It is a special centrifugate that can purify and satiate at the same time.

The diet's first stage has this much juice as its focal food, green because of its ingredients.

How to prepare green juice

Ingredients:
- 75g kale
- 30g rocket salad
- 5g parsley
- 2 celery sticks
- ½ green apple
- Juice of ½ lemon
- ½ teaspoon matcha green tea

It is prepared by centrifuging 75 grams of kale, 30 grams of rocket salad, and 5 grams of parsley.

Add 150 grams of green celery with leaves and half a green apple, both grated.

Finally, half squeezed lemon and half teaspoon of matcha tea will enrich the whole with antioxidants and vitamins.

This detox drink should preferably be prepared at the time of consumption, without storing it in the fridge, not to lose valuable benefits of the nutrients.

Options

If the taste is not pleasant, it is possible to make changes or add additional ingredients to make it tastier.

- ✓ Add a few mint leaves
- ✓ You can use a whole apple
- ✓ You can remove the parsley and add the strawberries
- ✓ You can drink water right after you drink it.
- ✓ It can be more pleasant cold, adding a little ice
- ✓ You can change the arugula with 1cm ginger

Recipes

Prawns with buckwheat

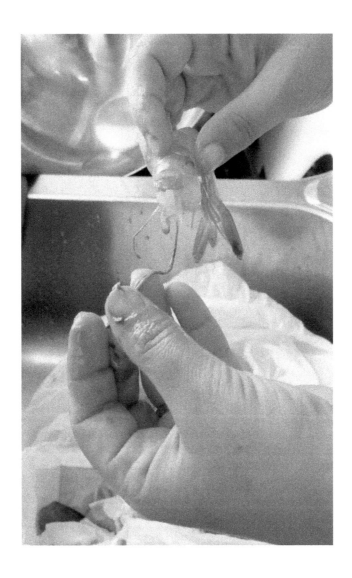

Serving 1

Ingredients:

- 150 g peeled prawns
- 1 teaspoon of tamari
- 2 teaspoons of extra virgin olive oil
- 75 g of buckwheat spaghetti
- 1 clove of garlic
- 1 chilli
- 1 teaspoon of ginger
- 20 g of red onion
- 40 g celery
- 75 g of chopped green beans,
- 50 g kale

Directions

1. Cook the shelled prawns for 2-3 minutes with one teaspoon of tamari and one teaspoon of extra virgin olive oil.
2. Boil the buckwheat spaghetti in water without salt, drain them and keep them aside.
3. Fry with another teaspoon of extra virgin olive oil, the clove of garlic, chilli pepper, and a teaspoon of finely chopped fresh ginger, sliced red onion celery, chopped green beans, and coarsely chopped kale.

4. Add 100 ml of water and bring to the boil leaving the vegetables to simmer while they are still crispy inside.
5. Add the prawns, spaghetti, and 5 g celery leaves, bring them back to the boil and serve.

Turkey with cauliflower couscous

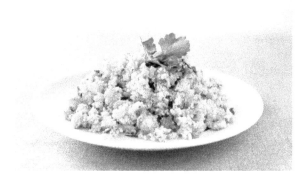

Serving 1

Ingredients:

- 150 g turkey
- 150 g of cauliflower tops
- 40 g of red onion
- 1 teaspoon of fresh ginger
- 1 Bird's-eye chilli
- 1 clove of garlic
- 3 teaspoons extra virgin olive oil
- 2 teaspoons of turmeric
- 30 g dried tomatoes
- 10 g parsley
- dried sage q.b.
- 1 tablespoon capers
- 1/4 fresh lemon juice

Directions

1. Blend the raw cauliflower tops and then cook them in a teaspoon of oil, garlic, red onion, chilli, ginger, and a teaspoon of turmeric, leave to flavor for a minute.

2. Add, over low heat, the chopped dried tomatoes and 5 g of parsley.

3. Season the turkey slice with one teaspoon of oil and the dried sage, and cook it in another teaspoon of oil.

4. Once ready, season with a tablespoon of capers, 1/4 of lemon juice, 5 g of parsley, a tablespoon of water, and add the cauliflower.

Chicken with red onion and kale

Serving 1

Ingredients:

- 120 g chicken breast
- 130 g of tomatoes
- 1 Bird's-eye chilli
- 1 tablespoon capers
- 5 g parsley
- lemon juice
- 2 teaspoons of extra virgin olive oil
- 2 teaspoons of turmeric
- 50 g kale
- 20 g of red onion
- 1 teaspoon of fresh ginger
- 50 g of buckwheat

Directions

1. Marinate the chicken breast for 10 minutes with 1/4 lemon juice, one teaspoon of oil, and one teaspoon of turmeric powder.

2. Cut 130 g of tomatoes into chunks, remove the inner part, season with chilli pepper, one tablespoon capers, 1 teaspoon turmeric and one teaspoon oil, juice of 1/4 lemon, and 5 g chopped parsley.

3. Cook the drained chicken breast over high heat for one minute on each side and then put it in the oven for about 10 minutes at 220°. Leave it to rest covered with aluminum foil.

4. Steam the chopped cabbage for 5 minutes; in a pan, fry the red onion, a teaspoon of freshly grated ginger, and a teaspoon of oil.

5. Add the boiled cabbage and leave to flavor together for one minute over the heat.

6. Boil the buckwheat with turmeric, drain and serve with chicken, tomatoes, and chopped cabbage.

Vegetable and buckwheat soup

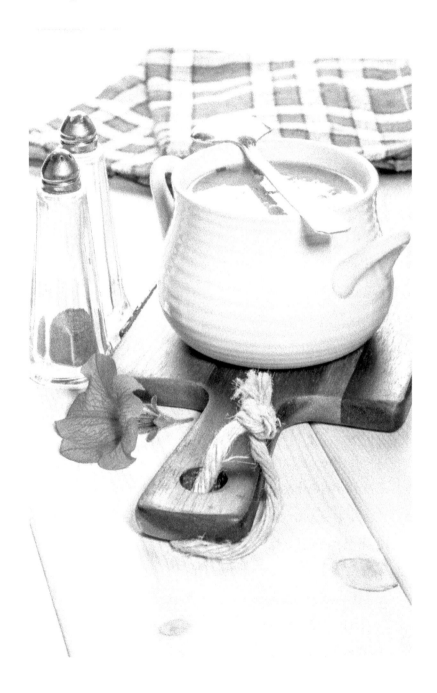

Serving 2

Ingredients:

- 200 g potatoes
- 200 g kohlrabi
- 100 g carrots
- 1 celery coast
- 1 red onion
- 500 ml of vegetable broth
- 1 tablespoon of extra virgin olive oil
- 2 cloves of garlic
- Halls
- 4 sage leaves
- 80 g of buckwheat
- 30 g of cheese
- 50 g of peeled red lentils

Directions

1. Wash the potatoes and kohlrabi, peel them, and cut them into cubes about an inch to the side.
2. Wash the carrots, peel them and slice them about 4 millimeters thick.
3. Wash the celery, remove the filaments and leaves, cut the rib into small cubes.
4. Peel the onion, cut it into quarters, then slice it to a thickness of 3-4 millimeters.
5. Heat the broth.

6. Put the oil and peeled garlic in a soup pot. Bring it to the heat and brown the garlic over a high flame.

7. Remove it, add all the vegetables, and cook, stirring for a couple of minutes.

8. Add the stock, keeping some aside for the end of cooking, a pinch of salt, the sage leaves well washed, put the lid on, and wait for it to boil.

9. Cook for 15 minutes after it starts boiling again over medium heat, covered.

10. After the indicated time, taste, and add salt regularly. The cooking stock must be a little tasty.

11. Rinse the buckwheat and lentils under freshwater, then add them to the pot.

12. Cook for 20 minutes over medium heat. Cook with the lid on if you want a more liquid soup, and without, if you want it thicker.

13. Al final, taste, and add salt regularly.

14. Turn off the heat, add the Parmesan cheese, stir well and let it rest, and covered for a couple of minutes. If the soup is too thick, add some of the stock set aside.

15. Serve with a drizzle of raw oil.

Pasta with smoked salmon, chilli, and rocket

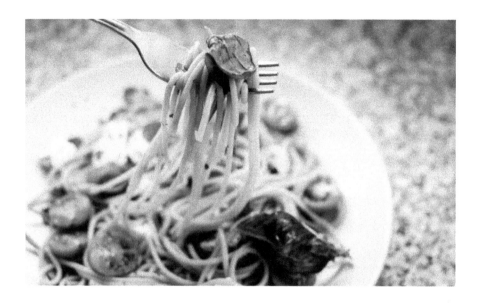

Serving: 4
Ingredients:

- 2 tablespoons of extra virgin olive oil
- 1 red onion, finely chopped
- 2 cloves of garlic, finely chopped
- 2 Bird's Eye chilli peppers, finely chopped
- 150g cherry tomatoes, cut in half
- 100ml white wine
- 250-300g buckwheat pasta
- 250g smoked salmon
- 2 tablespoons of capers

- 1/2 lemon juice
- 60g rocket salad
- 10g parsley, minced

Directions

1. Heat 1 teaspoon of oil in a pan over medium heat. Add the onion, garlic, and chilli, and fry until the ingredients are withered but not dark.
2. Add the tomatoes and leave to cook for a minute or two. Pour in the white wine and let it simmer until it reduces by half.
3. Cook the pasta in boiling water with one teaspoon of oil for 8-10 minutes, depending on whether you prefer it more or less al dente, and drain.
4. Cut the salmon into strips and transfer it to the tomato pot with capers, lemon juice, rocket, and parsley.
5. Add the pasta, stir well, and serve immediately. Sprinkle with any remaining oil.

Buckwheat and tofu salad

Ingredients

- 300 gr of buckwheat
- 400 gr of cherry tomatoes
- 125 gr of natural tofu
- 3 tufts of basil
- 150 gr of sunflower seeds
- Evo oil q.b.
- Salt q.b.

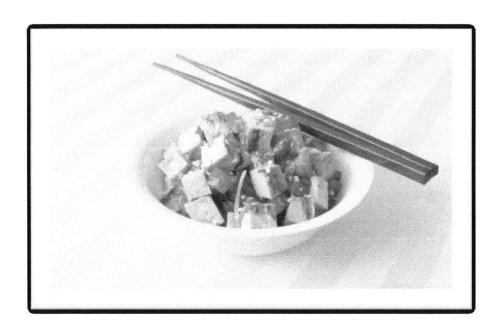

Directions

1. Rinse the buckwheat under running water, put it in a pot full of cold water, and cook for about twenty minutes; in the meantime, carefully wash the basil and tomatoes; cut the tomatoes into segments, and put them in a large bowl.

2. When cooked, drain the buckwheat, cool it under running water, then add it to the tomatoes; add the crumbled or chopped tofu, break up the basil and add the sunflower seeds. The season is fine with oil and salt, and mix everything.

3. You can also serve it immediately or after it has cooled well in the refrigerator.

4. *How to store tofu and buckwheat salad:*

5. You can store this salad in the refrigerator for a couple of days, but only if stored in airtight containers.

Chocolate Tartufini Sirt

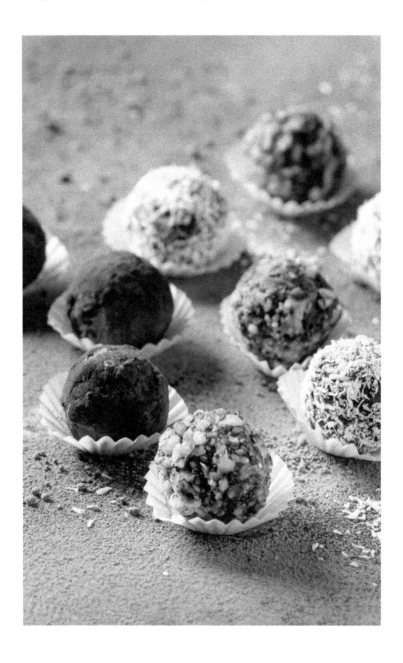

Ingredients for 15-20 truffles

- 120g walnuts
- 30g dark chocolate (85 percent cocoa), broken into pieces, or crushed cocoa beans
- 250g Medjoul dates, deprived of the seed
- 1 tablespoon of cocoa powder
- 1 tablespoon turmeric powder
- 1 tablespoon of extra virgin olive oil
- seeds of 1 vanilla pod or 1 teaspoon of vanilla extract
- 1-2 tablespoons of water

Directions:

1. Put the nuts and chocolate in a food processor and blend until a fine powder is obtained. Add all the other ingredients minus the water and blend until the mixture cures into a ball. You may have to add water, but it depends on the mix's consistency, which should not be too sticky.

2. Using your hands, form balls the size of walnuts and put them in the fridge in a sealed container for at least 1 hour before eating them. You can dip them in cocoa or dried coconut flakes to give them a slightly different taste. They will keep in the fridge for a week at most.

Sirt Salad

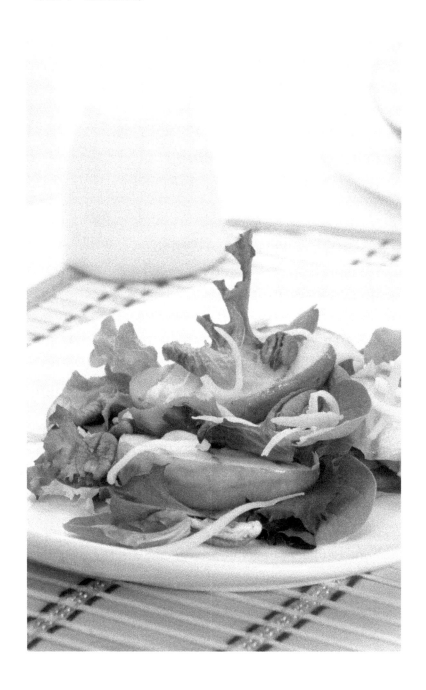

Ingredients:

- 1 portion 100g celery, coarsely chopped
- 50g apple, coarsely chopped
- 50g walnuts, coarsely chopped
- 10g red onion, coarsely chopped
- 5g chopped parsley
- 1 tablespoon capers
- 5g of lovage or celery leaves, coarsely chopped
- 1 tablespoon of extra virgin olive oil
- 1 tablespoon balsamic vinegar
- 1/4 lemon juice
- the tip of a teaspoon of Dijon mustard
- 50g arugula
- 35g red chicory leaves

Directions

1. Mix celery, apple, walnuts, onion, parsley, capers, and lovage or celery leaves. In a bowl, mix the oil, vinegar, lemon juice, and mustard and work everything with whips to obtain the seasoning.
2. Place the celery mixture on the rocket and red chicory and pour over the sauce.

Buckwheat pancakes with strawberries and chocolate

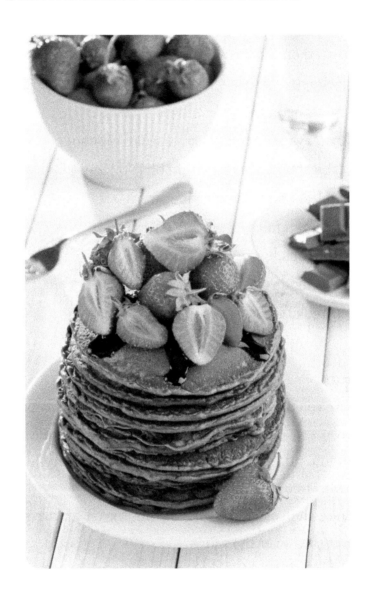

Ingredients for 6-8 pancakes

For pancakes

- 350ml of milk
- 150g buckwheat flour
- 1 big egg
- 1 tablespoon of extra virgin olive oil
- For the chocolate sauce:
- 100g dark chocolate (85 percent cocoa).
- 85ml of milk
- 1 tablespoon double cream
- 1 tablespoon of extra virgin olive oil

For garnish:

- 400g strawberries, peeled and chopped.
- 100g of chopped walnuts

Directions:

1. To prepare the pancakes, pour all the ingredients minus the oil into a blender and blend until the dough is smooth, not too dense, or too liquid. (You can store the excess in an airtight container in the refrigerator for up to 5 days. Make sure you mix it well before using it).
2. To prepare the sauce, melt the chocolate in a bowl on a pot of boiling water.

3. When it is melted, add the milk, stirring well, then the cream and olive oil. You can keep it warm by leaving it on the pot over a very low flame until the pancakes are ready.

4. Pour mixture into the pan, and move it by tilting it so that it is spread all over the surface. If necessary, add a little more of the mixture. It will take about a minute to cook on each side.

5. When the edges become brownish, use a spatula to lift the pancake along the outer perimeter and turn it.

6. Try to do this with a single movement to avoid breaking it. Cook it on the other side for a minute and transfer it to a tray.

7. Place some strawberries in the middle and roll up the pancake. Continue until you've made all the pancakes you want.

Pumpkin soup

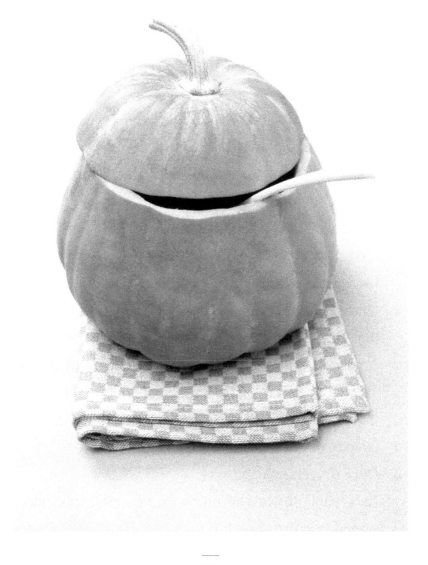

Serving: 4

Ingredients:

- 1500g pumpkin
- 1 tablespoon of miso
- 1 Lemon
- 1 Orange
- Red onion
- Extra virgin olive oil
- Salt q.b.

Directions

1. Choose a pumpkin with firm flesh.
2. Cut it into large pieces and put it directly into the oven without any seasoning.
3. Cook until soft (about 40 minutes at 180° in ventilated mode): in this way, the outer part will roast slightly and leave a great taste.
4. Once cooked, let it cool and then peel it. In the meantime, lower the oven to about 50 degrees.
5. Remove the peel (only the colored part, not the white skin) with half a lemon and about ¼ of orange - if you had a cedar, it would be even better - and put it in the oven to dry (about 10 minutes).
6. Once dry, chop it.
7. In a pan, brown the onion in vegetable oil; add the pumpkin pulp, stretch it with two glasses of water, and

blend it all. Add the citrus peel and a generous spoonful of miso. Let it simmer until the miso is melted and the ingredients mixed. Add salt and serve warm.

Chicken breast with walnut and parmesan pesto and red onion

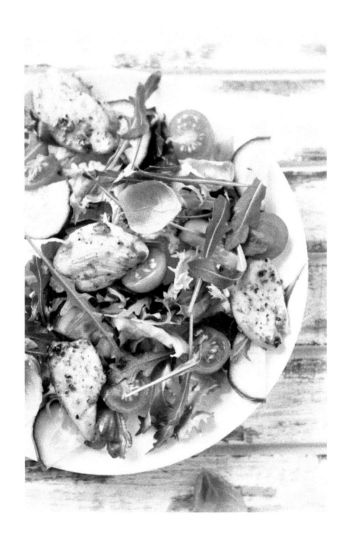

Serving 1

Ingredients:

- 15g parsley
- 15g pecans
- 4 teaspoons (15g) Parmesan cheese, minced
- 1 tablespoon of virgin olive oil
- 1/2 lemon juice
- 3 tablespoons (50ml) of water
- 150g chicken breast without the skin
- 20g red onions, finely chopped
- 1 teaspoon of red wine vinegar
- 35g rocket
- 100g split cherry tomatoes
- 1 teaspoon of balsamic vinegar

Directions:

1. Put the parsley, pecans, parmesan, parmesan, olive oil, most lemon juice, and some water in a food processor or blender and stir until smooth.

2. Include more water slowly until the desired consistency is obtained. Marinate the chicken breast in 1 tablespoon of pesto and the rest of the lemon juice in the cooler for 30 minutes; longer if possible.

3. Preheat the stove to 392°F (200°C).

4. Heat an oven-proof pan with medium to high heat.

5. Fry the marinated chicken on both sides, then move it to the oven, cook for 8 minutes, or fully cooked. Marinate the onions in red wine vinegar for 5-10 minutes.

6. When the chicken is cooked, remove it from the plate, put another spoonful of pesto on it and let the pesto melt with the chicken's heat.

7. Let it rest for 5 minutes before serving.

8. Add the rocket, tomatoes, onion, and sprinkle with balsamic vinegar.

Meat and chilli

Serving: 4

Ingredients:

- 1 red onion, finely chopped
- 3 cloves of garlic, finely chopped
- 2 Thai chilli peppers, finely chopped
- 1 tablespoon of additional virgin olive oil
- 1 tablespoon of ground cumin
- 1 tablespoon of ground turmeric
- 450g ground lean hamburger (5 percent fat)
- 150ml of red wine
- 1 chilli pepper, with core, semi-evacuated and cut into small pieces
- 400g jars of cut tomatoes
- 1 tablespoon of tomato puree
- 1 tablespoon of cocoa powder
- 150g canned beans
- 300ml meat broth
- 2 tablespoons (5g) of new, cut coriander
- 2 tablespoons (5g) fresh parsley, chopped
- 1 cup (160g) of buckwheat

Directions

1. In a huge pot, fry the onion, garlic, and bean stew in oil over medium heat for 2 or 3 minutes, including the flavors and cook for another moment or two.

2. Include the ground hamburger and cook for 2 or 3 minutes over medium-high heat until the meat is nicely caramelized everywhere. Include the red wine and let it rise to decrease significantly.

3. Add the red pepper, tomatoes, tomato puree, cocoa, beans, and broth, and leave to stew for 60 minutes.

4. You can include a little water from time to time to get a thick, sticky consistency.

5. Not long before serving, stir in the cut herbs. In the meantime, cook the buckwheat as indicated in the bundle guidelines and serve near the stew.

Pizza Sirt

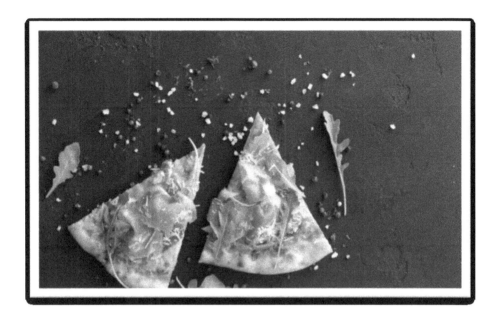

Ingredients:

(for two pizzas of 30cm)

For the pizza base:

- 1 pack of 7g dry yeast
- 1 teaspoon of brown sugar
- 300ml of lukewarm water
- 200g buckwheat flour
- 200g strong white flour or type 00
- 1 tablespoon of extra virgin olive oil, and a little more for oiling

For the tomato sauce:

- 1/2 red onion, finely chopped
- 1 clove of garlic, finely chopped
- 1 teaspoon of extra virgin olive oil
- 1 teaspoon of dried oregano
- 2 tablespoons of white wine
- 1 jar of 400g of tomato puree
- 1 pinch of brown sugar
- 5g basil leaves

Ideas for seals:

- Rocket, red onion, and grilled eggplant.

Directions

1. Heat a plate until it starts smoking, then reduce the temperature by adjusting the stove to a medium flame.
2. Slice eggplant in 3-5mm slices, brush them with a little extra virgin olive oil, and cook until you have black marks on both sides of the eggplant and the pieces are nice and soft.
3. Alternatively, you can bake it in the oven on a baking tray covered with baking paper, at 200°C, for 15 minutes, or until it is soft and well browned):
   a. Chilli flakes, cherry tomatoes, goat cheese, and arugula

b. Chicken already cooked, rocket, red onion, and olives

c. Cooked chorizo, red onion, and steamed kale

For the dough:

1. Dissolve the yeast and sugar in water: This will help activate the yeast. Sift the flour into a bowl. (If you have a food processor, put the kneading hook and pour the flour dough into the bowl provided).

2. Pour the yeast and oil mixture into the flour and knead. You may need to add a little water if the mix is too dry. Work until the mixture is homogeneous and elastic. Transfer it to an oiled bowl, cover with a clean damp cloth and leave to rise in a warm place for 45-60 minutes, until it has doubled in volume.

3. In the meantime, prepare the tomato sauce. Fry the onion and garlic in olive oil, then add the oregano. Add the wine and simmer until it reduces by half.

4. Add the tomato puree and sugar, bring to the boil and cook for 30 minutes until the sauce is thick. Break the basil leaves into pieces and add them to the sauce.

5. Heat the oven to 230°C (446°F).

6. Cut the dough in half and roll out both dough pieces on a pizza stone or non-stick baking sheet until the desired thickness is reached.

7. Spread a thin layer of tomato sauce on the surface (you only need half of the sauce for this amount of dough,

but you can freeze what remains), avoiding a fine strip along the edge. Add the rest of the ingredients (if you are using rocket and chilli flakes, add them after cooking).

8. Let it rest about 15-20 minutes before baking, so the dough will rise a little more, becoming lighter.
9. Bake in the oven for 10-12 minutes or until the cheese is golden brown.
10. If you use them, add the arugula and chilli flakes at the end of cooking.

Buckwheat pasta salad

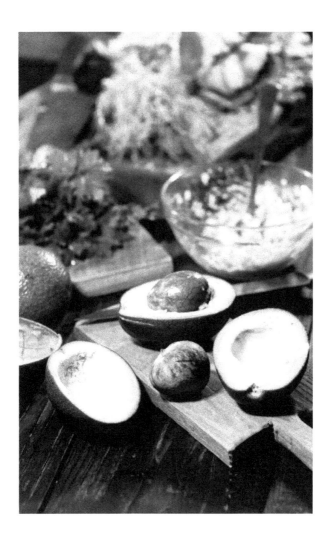

Ingredients:

- 50g of buckwheat pasta
- 1 large handful of arugula
- 1 handful of basil leaves
- 8 cherry tomatoes, cut in half
- 1/2 diced avocados
- 10 olives
- 1 tablespoon of extra virgin olive oil
- 20g pine nuts

Directions

1. Gently mix all the ingredients except the pine nuts, place them on a plate, and then spread them on top.

Buckwheat and broccoli with chickpeas

Serving 2

Ingredients:

- 100 g of buckwheat
- 150 g of cooked chickpeas
- 1 Roman cabbage
- 1 red onion
- 3 tablespoons of low-fat yogurt
- 1 cm of ginger root
- 2 tablespoons of extra virgin olive oil
- salt and pepper to taste
- 1 teaspoon of turmeric powder

Directions

2. Boil the cabbage florets in salted water for 10 minutes; in the meantime, toast the buckwheat (left to soak for a couple of hours) in a non-stick pan for about 5 minutes, then boil it in the cabbage cooking water (after draining them) for 15-20 minutes.

3. In a separate pan, fry the onion and ginger root in 2 tablespoons of oil, add the cabbage florets, the cooked chickpeas, and finally the buckwheat, letting it cook for a few minutes.

4. Turn it off, and if you like, accompany the dish with a yogurt sauce prepared by mixing the turmeric with the yogurt, adding a pinch of salt and pepper.

Buckwheat meatballs.

Serving 2/4

Ingredients:

- 100 grams of buckwheat;
- 1 whole egg;
- a clove of garlic;
- a bunch of parsley;
- nutmeg;
- breadcrumbs;
- salt and pepper.

Directions:

1. Wash the buckwheat and transfer it to a pot. Let it toast for a few seconds, after which add about 250/300 ml of cold water, add a pinch of salt, and cook for about 20-25 minutes.
2. Chop a clove of garlic and put it in a pan with a drizzle of oil
3. . Add the buckwheat well drained from the remaining cooking water and let it flavor together for a few minutes.
4. Transfer everything into a bowl and let it cool.
5. When the wheat is warm, add the slightly beaten egg, nutmeg, finely chopped parsley, a pinch of pepper, and mix well.

Cooking:

1. Now form some balls with the help of a spoon and roll them in breadcrumbs.

2. Compact the meatballs by squeezing them between the palms of your hands and, at the same time, flatten them slightly at the poles.

3. Grease a pan with oil and cook the meatballs on both sides until they are golden brown. Serve them hot buckwheat meatballs accompanied by vegetables to taste.

Cabbage and buckwheat fritters

Broccoli and buckwheat fritters are a tasty preparation for singles prepared by cooking the chopped shallot with broccoli in a pressure cooker. The buckwheat will be added at the end of cooking the mixture will be added to the flour.

The meatballs will be obtained crushed and will be fried, and served immediately on the table.

Ingredients:

- 20 g grated cheese
- 50 g cabbage tops
- 1 egg
- 1 tablespoon Flour 00
- 1/2 shallot
- Extra virgin olive oil
- Salt

Directions:

1. Clean the cabbage and choose the florets. Finely chop the shallot and put it in the pressure cooker with 1 tablespoon of oil and the cabbage florets.
2. Brown gently, add the buckwheat and twice as much saltwater or vegetable broth. Close the pan and cook for 15 minutes from the start of the hiss.

3. Open the pot and let the mixture cool down. Add the egg and add enough flour to obtain a homogeneous mixture with a moderately firm consistency.
4. If necessary, add salt to taste. With floured hands, form round meatballs and then crush them slightly to flatten them.
5. Place them in a baking tray and brush them with a drizzle of oil. Bake them in the oven for 15 minutes at about 200 °C (392 °F)

Buckwheat salad with artichokes

Serving: 4

Ingredients:

- 300 g buckwheat
- 200 g cherry tomatoes
- 5 artichokes
- 1 clove of garlic
- 1/2 cup large green olives
- fresh marjoram
- 5 tablespoons extra virgin olive oil
- salt
- 1 lemon

Directions:

1. In a non-stick pan, toast the buckwheat grains, always stirring for 3 or 4 minutes, then boil it in plenty of salted water for 10 minutes. It must remain very al dente. Drain and set aside.

2. Clean the artichokes: remove the outer leaves, trim them and remove the beard, cut them into segments, and throw them away as they are cleaned in water acidulated with lemon juice so that they do not blacken.

3. In the meantime, brown the clove of garlic dressed lightly crushed in two tablespoons of oil.

4. When the artichokes are all hulled and cut, drain them and put them in the pan. Brown them without burning,

then lower the heat and cook until they have softened a bit; they must remain al dente. Remove the garlic clove and sprinkle with a little fresh marjoram.

5. Put the buckwheat in the pan with the artichokes, stir well, and cook for a couple of minutes to make it taste good. Turn off and set aside.

6. Wash and cut the cherry tomatoes in half, leaving them a little in a colander to drain the vegetation water.

7. Cut the olives in half and remove the stone.

8. Incorporate the cherry tomatoes and olives with buckwheat, add more marjoram leaves, stir and let them flavor well covered over low heat.

Pasta with rocket salad and linseed

Serving: 4

Ingredients:

- 400 gr of wholemeal pasta
- 1 bunch of washed and dried Rocket
- 1 tablespoon of peeled almonds
- 1 tablespoon Linseed
- 1/2 clove of Garlic
- 4 spoons of extra virgin olive oil
- 3 tablespoons of water (if necessary)
- A few drops of lemon juice
- Salt
- Pepper

Directions:

1. First, wash the arugula and put it to dry on a kitchen cloth, then bring a pot of water to boil and throw the dough;
2. In a mixer, add 1 tablespoon of linseed, 1 tablespoon of almonds, half a clove of garlic (without the sprout), and 4 tablespoons of oil;
3. Cut everything for a few minutes, if necessary, add a little water to make the pesto more fluid;
4. At this point, add the rocket, a few drops of lemon juice, a pinch of salt and turn the mixer again for a few

seconds, then add salt and pepper, and your pesto is ready;

5. Before draining the pasta, set aside some cooking water so that it can be used later, in case the pesto is too thick;

6. Once drained, put the pasta on the pot, season it with the pesto, and, if necessary, add a little cooking water previously-stored, continuing to stir for about a minute, and now your dish is ready to taste!

Rocket and strawberry salad

Serving: 1

Ingredients

- 1 tuft of rocket
- 8 champignon mushrooms
- 12 strawberries
- 1 tablespoon of extra virgin olive oil
- half a teaspoon of mustard
- salt
- pepper
- lemon juice

Directions

1. Wash and dry the rocket, then break the leaves into a bowl. Clean and slice the mushrooms and 8 ripe and firm strawberries.
2. Also, put these ingredients in the bowl with the rocket. Mash 4 more strawberries well, add one tablespoon of extra virgin olive oil, half a teaspoon of mustard, salt, pepper, lemon juice, and emulsify with care.
3. Pour the sauce over the salad, stir and serve.

Sirt Meat & chilli

Serving: 4

Ingredients

- 1 red onion, finely chopped
- 3 cloves of garlic, finely chopped
- 2 Bird's Eye chilli peppers, finely chopped
- 1 tablespoon of extra virgin olive oil
- 1 tablespoon of cumin powder
- 1 tablespoon turmeric powder
- 400g of ground lean beef (5% fat)
- 150ml of red wine
- 1 red pepper deprived of the stalks and seeds and cut into pieces
- 2 jars of 400g of peeled tomatoes
- 1 tablespoon of tomato paste
- 1 tablespoon of cocoa powder
- 150g canned beans
- 300ml beef broth
- 5g of chopped coriander
- 5g chopped parsley
- 160g buckwheat

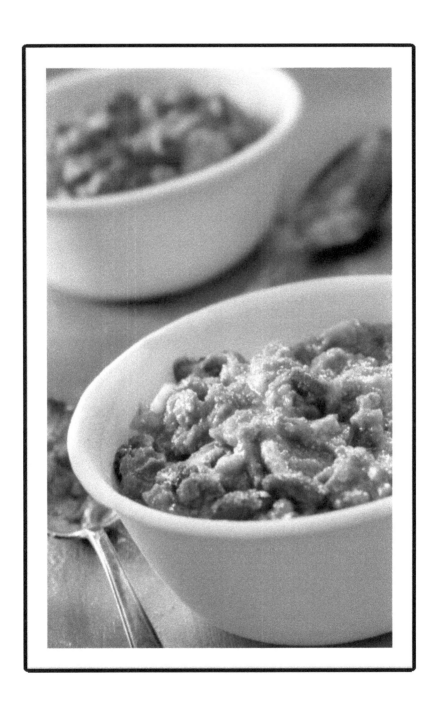

Directions

1. In a saucepan, fry onion, garlic, and chilli pepper in oil, over medium heat for 2-3 minutes. Add the spices and cook for another minute or two. Add the minced meat and cook for another 2 or 3 minutes over medium-high heat until well browned. Pour in the red wine and simmer until it reduces by half.

2. Add the pepper, peeled tomatoes, tomato paste, cocoa, beans, broth, and simmer for 1 hour.

3. You may have to add a little water from time to time to get a thick sweet sauce. Add the chopped herbs just before serving.

4. Cook the buckwheat according to the instructions on the package and serve with the chilli.

Sirt Eggs

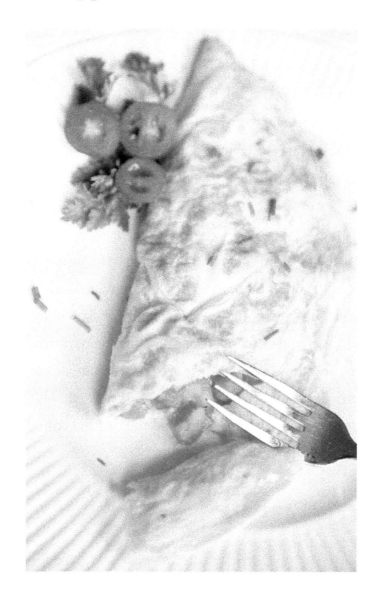

Serving: 1

Ingredients

- 1 teaspoon of extra virgin olive oil
- 20g red onion, finely chopped
- 1/2 Bird's Eye chilli, finely chopped
- 3 average eggs 50ml milk
- 1 teaspoon of turmeric powder
- 5g parsley, finely chopped

Directions

1. Heat the oil in a frying pan and fry the onion and chilli pepper until soft, but do not let them darken.
2. Beat the eggs, milk, turmeric, and parsley. Pour into the hot pan and cook over medium-low heat, move the eggs to scramble, and prevent them from sticking and burning.
3. Serve when you have obtained the desired consistency.

Sirt Yogurt

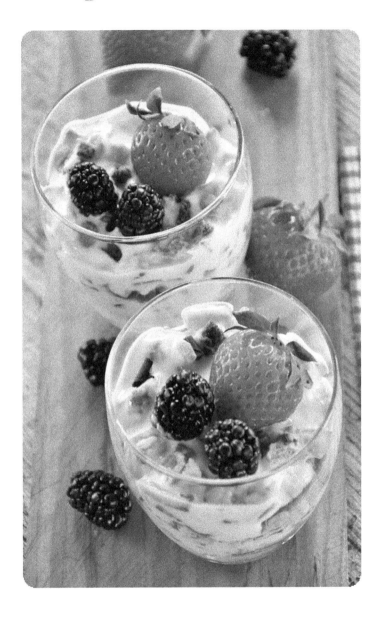

Serving: 1

Ingredients

- 125g mixed berries
- 150g Greek yogurt
- 25g of chopped walnuts
- 10g of dark chocolate (85 percent cocoa) grated

Directions

1. Put your favorite berries in a bowl and pour yogurt on top. Sprinkle them with nuts and chocolate.
2. For a vegan alternative, you can replace Greek yogurt with soy or coconut milk.

Sirt pita bread

Whole grain pitas are an excellent way to fill up your Sirt food in a practical, fast and easily transportable way. You can vary the quantities and have fun with the combinations, but the important thing is that you end up with a nice pita filled with excellent ingredients.

Ingredients
- 1 whole pita bread

Version with meat:
- 80g turkey sliced, minced
- 20g of diced Cheddar (or other cheese)
- 35g diced cucumbers
- 30g of chopped red onion
- 25g of chopped rocket
- 10-15g of coarsely chopped walnuts

For the sauce:
- 1 tablespoon of extra virgin olive oil
- 1 tablespoon balsamic vinegar
- a splash of lemon juice

Vegan version:
- 2-3 tablespoons of hummus
- 35g diced cucumbers

- 30g of chopped red onion
- 25g of chopped rocket
- 10-15g of coarsely chopped walnuts

Vegan sauce:
- 1 tablespoon of extra virgin olive oil
- a splash of lemon juice

Sirt Omelette

Serving: 1

Ingredients:

- 50g striped bacon (smoked or natural, according to taste)
- 3 medium eggs
- 35g red radicchio, finely sliced
- 5g parsley, finely chopped
- 1 teaspoon of extra virgin olive oil

Directions

1. Warm-up a non-stick frying pan. Cut the bacon into strips and fry it over a high flame until crispy—no need to add oil, just the bacon fat.

2. Remove from the heat and place it on a sheet of kitchen paper to dry the excess fat. Clean the pan.

3. Beat the eggs and add the radicchio and parsley. Cut up the fried bacon and add it to the eggs.

4. Heat the oil in the non-stick pan, which should be hot, but not steaming.

5. Add the egg mixture and, using a spatula, move them to obtain smooth cooking. Reduce the flame and let the omelet harden. Lift it along the edges with the wooden spatula, fold it in half, or roll it up and serve.

Red bean sauce with baked potato

Serving: 1

Ingredients:

- 40g red onion, finely chopped
- 1 teaspoon of fresh ginger, finely chopped
- 1 clove of garlic, finely chopped
- 1 Bird's Eye chilli pepper, finely chopped
- 1 teaspoon of extra virgin olive oil
- 1 teaspoon of turmeric powder
- 1 teaspoon of cumin powder
- 1 pinch of powdered cloves
- 1 pinch of cinnamon powder
- 1 medium potato 190g peeled
- 1 teaspoon of brown sugar
- 50g red pepper, stripped of stalks and seeds and coarsely chopped
- 150ml vegetable stock
- 1 tablespoon of cocoa powder
- 1 teaspoon of sesame seeds
- 2 teaspoons of peanut butter (the velvety one is better, but the crunchy one is fine too)
- 150g canned red beans
- 5g chopped parsley

Directions

1. Heat the oven to 200 °C (392 °F).

2. Fry the onion, ginger, garlic, and chilli pepper in oil in a medium pan over medium heat for about 10 minutes or until the ingredients have withered. Add the spices and cook for another 1-2 minutes.

3. Place the potato on a baking tray, put it in the hot oven, and cook for 45-60 minutes until it is soft on the inside (or even longer if you like it crunchy on the outside).

4. Add the peeled tomatoes, sugar, peppers, stock, cocoa powder, sesame seeds, peanut butter, beans, and simmer for 45 to 60 minutes.

5. Finally, sprinkle with parsley.

Tuna turkey

For Vegetable Bouillon:

- 2 potatoes
- 1 red onion
- 2 carrots
- 1 celery stalk
- Salt
- Pepper
- 1 tablespoon Extra virgin olive oil

For the meat:

- 800g Turkey breast
- 1 carrot
- 1 celery
- ½ red onion
- 1 bay leaf
- Juniper berries
- Salt
- Pepper
- 1 rosemary sprig

For the tuna sauce:

- 200g canned tuna
- 2 eggs
- 5 anchovy fillets

- 1 tablespoon capers

Directions

The tuna turkey, also called tonnè, is a second meat dish very simple to prepare. We use turkey meat, less fatty, but still very tasty. The homemade tuna sauce softens the turkey giving it an unmistakable texture and flavor. Follow the recipe step by step, and you will prepare an alternative dish to enjoy with your family.

1. Prepare the vegetable stock. Coarsely cut a carrot, a peeled potato, a celery rib, and an onion with a drizzle of oil, a pinch of salt, and pepper.
2. Leave to cooking for 10 minutes after boiling, then lower the heat to a minimum.
3. Prepare the vegetables to cook with the meat: cut a carrot, an onion, and a celery rib. Take the turkey breast and tie it with a sprig of rosemary, helping yourself with a string as if it were a roast.
4. In a large pan, put the turkey to brown in oil with the cut vegetables, a bay leaf, some juniper berries, and a pinch of salt and pepper. Let it brown on all sides turning it gently. At this point, blend with the white wine and let it evaporate.
5. Completely cover the meat and vegetables with the broth and close the pan with a lid. Leave to cook for an hour over gentle heat until the soup has dried, turn off, and let the meat rest.

6. Remove the turkey string, slice it with a knife into slices of about one centimeter. Cover them with the tuna sauce. Garnish the turkey with some capers and enjoy it.

Tips
You can store your tuna turkey for up to three days in the fridge.

Stew with sirtfood

Serving: 6

Ingredients:

- 1.2 kg beef
- 200 ml red wine
- 80 gr tomato paste
- 4 tablespoons extra virgin olive oil
- 2 garlic cloves
- 1 carrot
- 1 red onion
- 1 celery ribs
- 1 clump of sage
- 1 rosemary sprig
- Broth
- Salt
- Pepper
- Kitchen twine

Directions

1. The cooking of this recipe is long, but the scents that will be released at home will be worth every wait. Chop the garlic with rosemary and sage until you have a finely chopped.

2. Make small cuts on the meat and use your fingers to insert the chopped meat to flavor the meat. Tie the

meat with string so that it keeps its shape while cooking.

3. Pour the oil and the rest of the chopped vegetables into a saucepan. Insert the piece of meat and brown it slightly. Blend in the red wine and let the alcohol evaporate.

4. Add the tomato paste. Lower the heat and cook for about 3 hours, until the vegetables are chopped and the meat is very soft.

5. Add salt and pepper and serve piping hot.

Curly kale with sweet potatoes

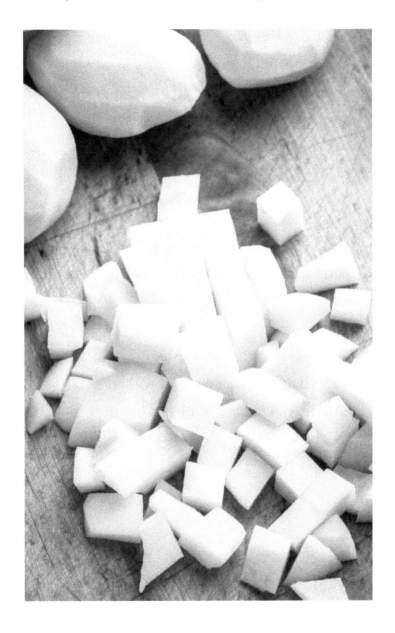

Serving: 1

Ingredients:

- 50g Curly Kale
- 200 g Sweet potatoes
- Red onion
- 1 teaspoon bird's eye chilli pepper
- 2 tablespoons extra virgin olive oil
- Salt

Directions

1. Cut the sweet potatoes into small cubes and put them in a pan with a drizzle of oil and the onion into small pieces.
2. Add salt.
3. Once cooked, add the cut kale and chilli pepper.
4. Turn well until the kale is well withered.
5. Continue cooking for another 5 minutes, always stirring with a ladle!

Buckwheat pasta with zucchini and cherry tomatoes

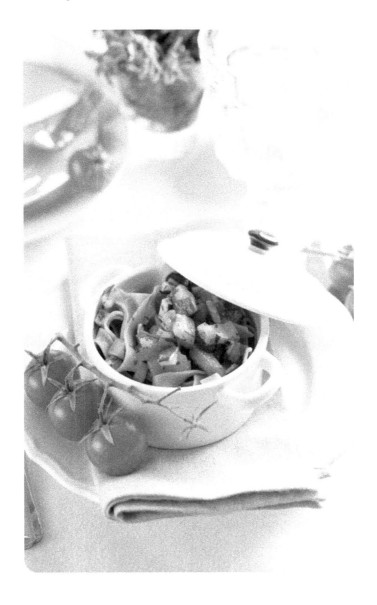

Serving: 2

Ingredients:

- 160 g buckwheat pasta
- 2 zucchini
- 6 cherry tomatoes
- 1/2 red onion
- extra virgin olive oil
- halls
- bird's-eye chilli

Directions

1. Fry the oil in a pan with the sliced onion and chilli pepper.
2. When the onion has taken a little color, add the cherry tomatoes and zucchini slices; turn well and let cook with a lid on medium heat for about 10 minutes, turning occasionally.
3. Boil the water for the pasta, add salt and drain the pasta.
4. Throw it directly into the sauce and fry everything in a pan for about a minute.

Chicken curry with potatoes and cabbage

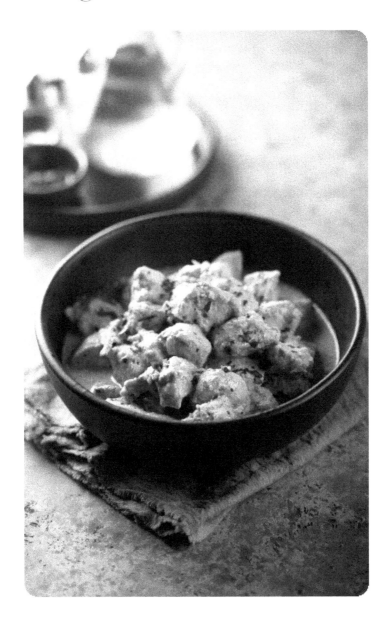

Serving: 4

Ingredients:

- 600g chicken breast, cut into pieces
- 4 tablespoons of extra virgin olive oil
- 3 tablespoons of turmeric
- 1 red onion, sliced
- 2 red chili peppers, finely chopped
- 2 cloves of garlic, finely chopped
- 1 tablespoon of freshly chopped ginger
- 1 tablespoon curry powder
- 1 jar of cherry tomatoes (400ml)
- 500ml chicken broth
- 200ml of coconut milk
- 2 pieces of cardamom
- 1 cinnamon stick
- 600g potatoes (mostly waxy)
- 10g parsley,
- 175g of kale, cut into pieces,
- 5g of chopped coriander

1. Marinate the chicken in a teaspoon of olive oil and a tablespoon of turmeric for about 30 minutes.
2. Fry it in a high frying pan over high heat for about 5 minutes. Remove from the pan and set aside.

3. Heat a tablespoon of oil in a pan with chilli, garlic, onion, and ginger. Boil over medium heat and then add the curry powder and a tablespoon of turmeric and cook for another minute, stirring occasionally.

4. Add the tomatoes, cook for another two minutes until the chicken stock, coconut milk, cardamom, and cinnamon stick are added.

5. Cook for about 45-60 minutes and add a little broth if necessary. Meanwhile, preheat the oven to 220 °C (425 °F).

6. Peel and chop the potatoes. Bring the water to a boil, add the potatoes with turmeric and cook for 3 minutes.

7. Remove them from the water and, in a baking tray, season them with olive oil and curry.

8. Bake in the oven for 30 minutes. When the potatoes and curry are almost ready, add the coriander, cabbage, and chicken and cook for 5 minutes until the chicken is hot.

9. Add the parsley to the potatoes and serve with the chicken curry.

Cabbage and buckwheat soup

Serving: 1

Ingredients:

- 1 teaspoon of extra virgin olive oil
- 1 teaspoon of mustard seeds
- 1 /4 cup (40g) red onion, finely chopped
- 2 cloves of garlic, finely chopped
- 1 teaspoon of finely chopped fresh ginger
- 1 Thai chili pepper, finely chopped
- 1 teaspoon of sweet curry powder, if you prefer)
- 2 teaspoons of ground turmeric
- 300ml vegetable stock or water
- 1 /4 cup (40g) Red Lentils, Rinsed
- 3 /4 cup (50g) kale, minced
- 50ml canned coconut milk
- 1 /3 cup (50g) buckwheat

Directions:

1. Heat the oil in a medium-sized saucepan over medium heat and add the mustard seeds. When the mustard seeds begin to pop, add the onion, garlic, ginger, and chilli pepper.
2. Cook for a few minutes.
3. Add the curry powder and one teaspoon of turmeric.

4. After a couple of minutes, add lentils in a pan and broth.
5. Bring to the boil over low heat for another 25-30 minutes, until they are cooked thoroughly.
6. Add the kale and coconut milk and cook for another 5 minutes.   In the meantime, cook the buckwheat according to the package instructions with the remaining teaspoon of turmeric. Drain it and serve it next to the cabbage and lentil soup.

Pasta with red chicory and walnuts

Serving: 1

Ingredients:

- 70 g buckwheat pasta
- 100 g red chicory
- 10 g extra virgin olive oil
- 20 g walnuts
- 30 g bacon cut into strips
- 10g Bird's eye chili minced
- Salt

Directions:

1. Stew the red chicory in a saucepan with oil.
2. When cooked, add the walnut grains you have previously browned with bacon cut into strips.
3. In another pot, cook the pasta in salted water, drain it, add it to the mixture of red chicory and walnuts and sauté for a few seconds.
4. At final, a sprinkling of chili.

Cabbage and red chicory flan

Serving: 4

Ingredients:

- 800g cabbage
- 250g red chicory
- 100g red onions 100 g
- 3 tablespoons Extra virgin olive oil
- Salt
- Pepper
- 2 tablespoon breadcrumbs
- 60g walnuts

Directions

1. Clean the cauliflower by eliminating the green leaves and the central core, and always with the help of a smooth blade knife, detach all the tops, dividing in half the bigger ones. Transfer the cleaned buds into a colander and rinse them under cold water.

2. Put a saucepan full of water on the fire and as soon as it boils, dip the cauliflower tops, cooking them for about 10 minutes; the consistency will have to remain rather al dente since it will be sautéed in the pan; then continue with the cooking in the oven. Drain the cauliflower into a bowl and leave it aside.

3. Heat a drizzle of oil in a large pan, add the onion and sauté over low heat. As soon as the onion is golden, add the cauliflower, salt, and pepper to taste. Stir and let everything season for about 5-6 minutes.

4. In the meantime, clean the red chicory by removing the central core, slice it thinly, add it to the pan with the cauliflower, stir, and fry for a few seconds to not wither too much.

5. Put out the fire and set it aside. Chop the nuts.

6. Heat the oven to 200 °C in static mode. Grease 4 bowls with a diameter of about 11 cm and fill them with cauliflower and red chicory, sprinkle on the surface a pinch of breadcrumbs and walnut grains.

7. Bake for about 15 minutes, gratinating the last minutes of cooking with the grill to brown the surface. Remove from the oven and serve hot.

8. You can store the flan in a food container for 2-3 days. We do not recommend freezing.

Red chicory and kale salad

Serving: 4

Ingredients:

- 200 g of canned chickpeas
- 1 kale
- 1 red chicory
- 1 red onion
- 40g extra virgin olive oil
- Salt
- Lemon juice
- Walnuts
- Rocket salad

Directions

1. Clean the kale leaves and cut them into strips. Let them wither with finely chopped red onion in a non-stick pan with two tablespoons of extra virgin olive oil.

2. When the kale is cooked, mix it with the chickpeas, drained from their preserving liquid, in a salad bowl. The ingredient that will give that bitterish touch to the dish will be the red chicory, to be used raw.

3. Mix the various components and then season with fine salt, good extra virgin olive oil, and a splash of lemon, which will give acidity to the dish.

4. Add the walnuts and some arugula leaves to provide color and... enjoy your meal!

Salmon and rocket fusilli

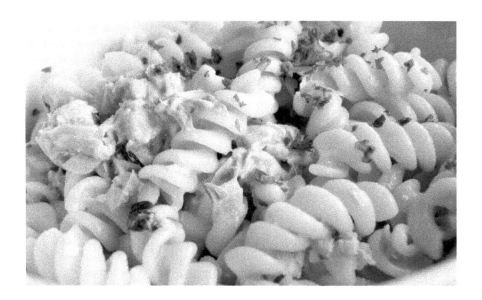

Serving: 4

Ingredients:

- 400 g of buckwheat fusilli
- 150 g salmon
- 30 g of fresh ginger
- 80 g arugula
- 1 clove of garlic
- extra virgin olive oil
- Salt
- bird's-eye chili

Directions

1. To prepare the rocket, salmon and ginger fusilli, put a pot of salted water on the fire. While the pasta is cooking, start making the sauce. Chop the arugula very finely and set it aside. Cut the salmon into cubes and brown it in a pan with a drizzle of oil and crushed garlic until it flakes.

2. Add the rocket, a few pieces of chili pounded in a mortar, salt, and ginger. Let it all season by stirring. Drain the fusilli well al dente and sauté them in the pan with the seasoning, adding a little cooking water.

3. Transfer the rocket, salmon, and ginger fusilli to the serving plates and serve immediately.

Cabbage soup and chickpeas with turmeric

The cabbage and chickpea soup with turmeric is an excellent first course that will warm you up in the autumn season. Thanks to vegetables and legumes, healthy and nutritious, it is also suitable for those who follow a vegetarian diet.

Coconut milk, so delicate in flavor, harmonizes very well with white cauliflower with a stronger taste, while chickpeas, partly smoothies, give the cream a particular body. Finally, the ginger provides the dish with a spicy note just lively that warms and regenerates, while the turmeric completes the dish with color.

Ingredients:

Serving: 4

- 1 cabbage
- 250 g of chickpeas already cooked
- 400 ml of coconut milk
- 2 teaspoons of turmeric powder
- 1 red onion
- 1 clove of garlic
- 3 cm of freshly grated ginger
- 400 ml hot water

- chopped parsley
- extra virgin olive oil
- salt
- bird's-eye chili

Directions

1. To prepare the cabbage and chickpea soup with turmeric, start by finely chopping the onion. Brown it in a saucepan with the oil and crushed garlic clove.

2. Add the turmeric, grated ginger, and stir in the onion and let it flavor for a couple of minutes. Add the coconut milk and bring to a boil.

3. Add the cabbage, cover with water, and cook until tender. Add the chickpeas and let them season for a few minutes. Fill half of the soup to obtain a cream and stir in salt and chilli.

4. Transfer the cauliflower and chickpeas soup with turmeric to the serving plates and serve with fresh chopped parsley and a round of raw oil to taste.

Strawberries in salad

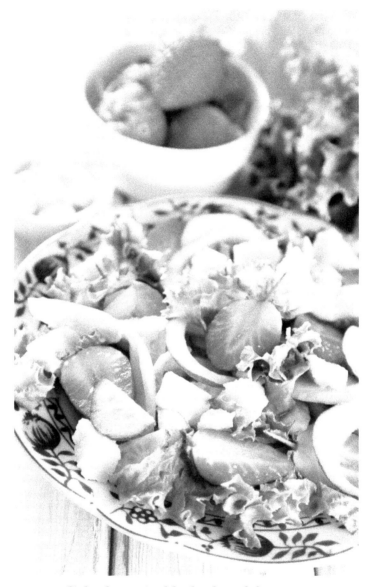

A great dish also suitable for breakfast

Serving: 4

Ingredients:

- 1 head of curly salad
- 150 g strawberries
- 150 g of mixed salads (rocket and soncino)
- extra virgin olive oil
- balsamic vinegar
- salt
- bird's-eye chilli

Directions

1. Wash and dry the strawberries, remove the stalks, and cut them into slices.
2. Wash the salads, dry them, chop them with your hands.
3. In a salad bowl, pick strawberries and vegetables, stir gently.
4. In a bowl, emulsify five tablespoons of oil, two balsamic vinegar, a pinch of salt, and a few chillies. Drizzle the salad with the sauce, stir and serve.

Turmeric chicken

Serving: 4

Ingredients:

- 4 chicken legs
- 4 tablespoons of flour
- 2 tablespoons of turmeric
- 1 red onion
- 20g extra virgin olive oil
- 200 ml of milk
- 4 teaspoons of mustard
- 150 ml of red wine

Directions

1. Flour the chicken with all powders (keeping a spoonful of turmeric aside).
2. In a frying pan, cook the sliced onion in oil. Add the chicken and brown it on both sides for a few minutes.
3. After the red wine has faded, add the milk in which you have dissolved the remaining turmeric.
4. Cook for 30-40 minutes before removing from the heat.
5. Add, if you like, mustard. As for the cooking of the chicken, adjust according to the size and quality of the meat.

Pork tenderloin with apricots

Serving: 4
Ingredients:

- 800 gr pork fillet
- 160 gr basmati rice
- 8 apricot
- 3 red onions
- 3 thyme twigs
- 1 rosemary sprig
- 1 teaspoon turmeric
- 2 tablespoons apple vinegar
- 7 tablespoons extra virgin olive oil
- Worcester sauce
- salt
- pepper

Directions

1. Boil 160 g of basmati rice in plenty of boiling salted water for about 10-12 minutes (or for the time indicated on the package) and drain it al dente.
2. Place it in a bowl and smell it with 1 teaspoon of turmeric.

3. Put in a glass jar 6 tablespoons of extra virgin olive oil, two tablespoons of apple vinegar, salt, and pepper, close with the lid, and shake vigorously to emulsify.

4. Prepare the other ingredients. While the rice is boiling, peel two red onions, cut them into large slices, cook them on the grill for 5 minutes on each side, arrange them in a baking dish and keep them warm in the oven at 180° C.

5. Wash, dry, and cut eight apricots in half without the stone, and cook them on the grill for 5 minutes on each side. Also, transfer the apricots to the baking tray.

6. Cut 800 g of pork fillet into 2.5 cm thick slices to make the meat tastier; leave the slices to rest for 20 minutes in a marinade made with one tablespoon of extra virgin olive oil, chopped onion, thyme, rosemary, and Worchestershire sauce.

7. Complete and serve. Cook the meat on the steak for about 6 minutes on each side. If needed, transfer the slices to a heat-resistant serving plate and keep them warm for a few minutes in the oven. When everything is ready, season the ingredients with the apple vinegar vinaigrette and serve at the table, accompanying the apricot pork tenderloin with the turmeric-scented rice.

Conclusion

We are sure you are delighted with the recipes in this book. As you have already observed, we have chosen tasty recipes that can be adapted to the entire family. In addition to being light, they will satisfy the most demanding palates!

Since this book is intended for international distribution, we thought it appropriate to include conversion tables from Grams to Ounces and Celsius to Fahrenheit degrees. So, are you ready to try all of our recipes? Enjoy!

Conversions

Grams to Ounces

1 gram (g) is equal to 0.03527396195 ounces (oz).

Formula:

g = 0.03527396195 oz

The mass y in ounces (oz) is equal to the mass y in grams (g) divided by 28.34952:

$$y_{(oz)} = y_{(g)} / 28.34952$$

Example

Convert 100g to Ounces:

$$y_{(oz)} = 100 \text{ g} / 28.34952 = 3,5274 \text{ oz}$$

Table

Grams (g)	Ounces (oz)
0 g	0 oz
1 g	0.0353 oz
2 g	0.0706 oz
3 g	0.1058 oz
4 g	0.1411 oz
5 g	0.1764 oz
6 g	0.2116 oz
7 g	0.2469 oz
8 g	0.2822 oz
9 g	0.3175 oz
10 g	0.3527 oz
20 g	0.7055 oz
30 g	1.0582 oz
40 g	1.4110 oz
50 g	1.7637 oz
60 g	2.1164 oz
70 g	2.4692 oz
80 g	2.8219 oz
90 g	3.1747 oz
100 g	3.5274 oz
1000 g	35.2740 oz

Celsius to Fahrenheit

0 grade Celsius (°C) is equal to 32 Fahrenheit (°F)
1 grade Celsius (°C) is equal to 33.8 F Fahrenheit (°F)
Formula:

$$n \,°C \times 9/5) + 32 = n \,°F$$

Example

Convert 200 °C to °F
(200 x 9/5)+32= 392 °F

Table

Celsius (°C)	Fahrenheit (°F)
0	32
60	140
70	158
80	176
90	194
100	212
110	230
120	248
130	266
140	284
150	302
160	320
170	338
180	356
190	374
200	392
210	410
220	428

Lightning Source UK Ltd.
Milton Keynes UK
UKHW020636020321
379651UK00008BA/161